ILLUSTRATED
OPERATION NOTES

A Guide for Students to General Surgical Procedures

Stephen Whitehead MChir FRCS

Senior Surgical Registrar St Thomas' Hospital

Edward Arnold

A division of Hodder & Stoughton

LONDON   BALTIMORE   AUCKLAND   MELBOURNE

© 1988 Stephen Whitehead

First published in Great Britain in 1988

British Library Catologuing in Publication Data

Whitehead, Stephen
   Illustrated operation notes : a guide for
   students to general surgery procedures
   1. Surgery, operative
   I. Title
   617'.91   RD32

   ISBN 0-340-41767-6

Whilst the advice and information in this book is believed to be true and accurate at the time of going to press, neither the authors nor the publisher can accept any legal responsibility or liability for any errors or omissions that may be made.

Typeset in Singapore by Colset Private Limited
Printed and bound in Great Britain for
Edward Arnold, the educational, academic and medical publishing division of Hodder & Stoughton Limited, 41 Bedford Square, London WC1B 3DQ
by Biddles Ltd, Guildford and King's Lynn

Contents

Preface

It is not at all difficult to grasp the concept of excision of an abdominal organ, be it the spleen, kidney or the humble appendix. It is rather more of a task, however, to understand the re-routeing of the gastrointestinal tract that takes place in, for example, a partial gastrectomy or a Whipple's operation.

I have not attempted to make a comprehensive list of operations, nor is this a guide to operative surgery. The operations I have described are those in which an element of 're-plumbing' is performed, and are those carried out by general surgeons. I have included small sections on some vascular and urological procedures that one might see in a District General Hospital.

I hope that this book will be used to clarify such procedures for all those involved in the care of patients, both in theatre and on the wards. It is particularly dedicated to those who have to decipher poorly written and badly drawn operation notes, or whose view of an operation in the theatre is obscured by bulky surgeons. The diagrams might also be useful in helping a patient understand his operation. A basic knowledge of anatomy is assumed, though a small glossary of unfamiliar terms has been included.

The book owes its inspiration to my wife Deborah. I am very grateful to her for her many suggestions and for the encouragement that she has offered.

Stephen Whitehead
London 1988

Note: Legends to figures

As in almost all cases, the figures illustrating an operation appear opposite the operation title and notes, it was not felt necessary to repeat the title of the operation next to the figure number as a legend. However, occasionally, descriptive or additional information has been supplied to qualify the illustration and this has been included next to the figure number.

GASTRODUODENUM
Truncal Vagotomy and Pyloroplasty

Indications

Duodenal ulcer.

Operative details

The anterior and posterior vagus nerves are divided proximal to the gastro-oesophageal junction. A segment of nerve is usually excised for histological confirmation.

The pylorus is enlarged by means of a longitudinal incision which is then sewn up transversely. There are other methods of pyloroplasty (e.g. Finney) that achieve the same effect. (See Figure 1).

Notes

Division of the trunks of the vagi interrupts the parasympathetic nerve supply to the whole of the stomach. Whilst this reduces acid secretion, denervation of the antrum and pylorus leads to failure of the stomach to empty. This is corrected by the pyloroplasty. Truncal vagotomy also interrupts the nerve supply to the rest of the gut and may result in troublesome diarrhoea. *Highly selective vagotomy* is without these complications.

Chronic ulceration may leave the pylorus so scarred and narrowed (pyloric stenosis) that a *gastroenterostomy* may be an easier method of creating adequate gastric drainage.

Truncal Vagotomy and Pyloroplasty

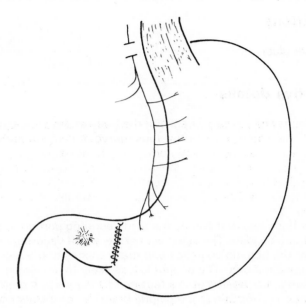

Fig. 1(a)   Only one vagus nerve shown for clarity

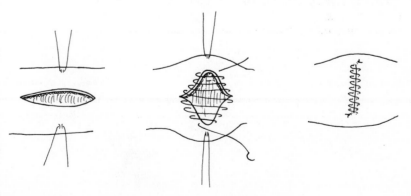

Fig. 1(b)   Detail of Heineke Mikulicz pyloroplasty

Highly Selective Vagotomy

Indications

Duodenal ulcer.

Operative details

The branches of the vagi supplying the body of the stomach are divided. The main trunk of the vagus (nerve of Laterjet) and the branches to the antrum and pylorus are left intact. (See Figure 2).

Notes

Only the branches that supply the acid-secreting portion of the stomach are divided. The selective nature of the vagotomy is such that the hepatic branches and the branches to the rest of the gut remain intact. The patient is less likely to develop the troublesome diarrhoea that is a feature of *truncal vagotomy*. Preservation of the antral and pyloric branches of the vagus allows the stomach to empty normally, obviating the need for a pyloroplasty.

The operation is more difficult and time-consuming than a *truncal vagotomy and pyloroplasty*, especially in an obese patient.

Highly Selective Vagotomy

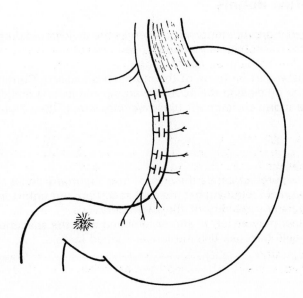

Fig. 2   Only one vagus nerve shown for clarity

Truncal Vagotomy and Antrectomy

Indications

Duodenal ulcer.

Operative details

The anterior and posterior vagus nerves are divided proximal to the gastro-oesophageal junction. A segment of nerve is usually excised for histological confirmation.

The distal part (antrum) of the stomach is excised. Continuity is restored by closing the duodenal stump and joining the jejunum onto the stomach remnant (*gastrojejunostomy*). (See Figure 3).

Notes

This procedure combines the effects of a *vagotomy* and a *gastrectomy* in reducing gastric acid secretion, but unfortunately combines the morbidity of the two operations.

The ulcer may be left *in situ* or removed with the specimen. If left, it heals because it is no longer bathed in acid.

Truncal Vagotomy and Antrectomy

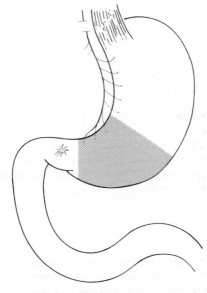

Fig. 3(a)   Only one vagus nerve shown for clarity

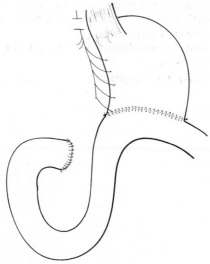

Fig. 3(b)   Reconstruction

13

Polya Gastrectomy

Indications

Duodenal ulcer.
High gastric ulcer.
Carcinoma of the stomach.

Operative details

The distal four-fifths of the stomach is removed. After closure of the duodenal stump (often leaving the ulcer *in situ*), continuity is restored by anastomosing the remains of the stomach (a) to the jejunum (b). (See Figure 4).

Notes

This reduces acid secretion by excision of all of the gastrin-producing cells (the antrum) and some of the acid-producing cells. Following reduction of acid secretion and diversion of acid away from the duodenum, the ulcer heals.

There is a higher complication rate than for *vagotomy*, but a lower chance of recurrence of a duodenal ulcer.

When performed for gastric ulcer or carcinoma, the lesion is removed in the resected part.

The operation was first performed by Billroth and is sometimes called a Billroth II operation.

Polya was a Hungarian surgeon.

Polya Gastrectomy

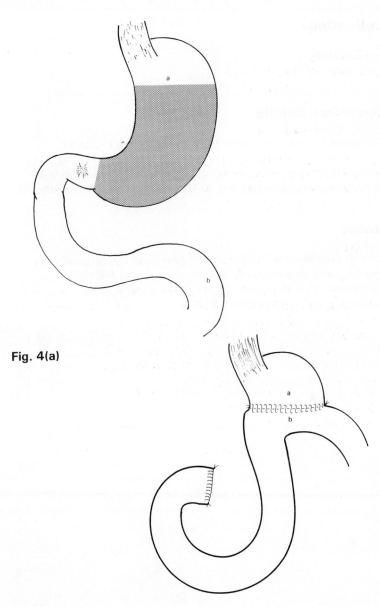

Fig. 4(a)

Fig. 4(b)   Reconstruction

Billroth I Gastrectomy

Indications

Gastric ulcer.
Carcinoma of the stomach.

Operative details

The distal stomach together with the ulcer are removed.
Continuity is restored by closing the gastric remnant along the
line a-b to form a 'new' lesser curve, and anastomosing the
remainder along the line b-c to the duodenum. (See Figure 5).

Notes

Billroth described another form of gastrectomy, originally for
carcinoma of the stomach, known now as the Billroth II
gastrectomy. It is similar to the *Polya gastrectomy*.
  Billroth was a Viennese surgeon.

Billroth I Gastrectomy

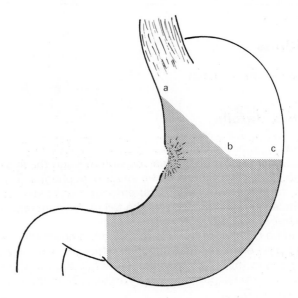

Fig. 5(a)

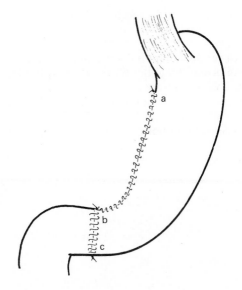

Fig. 5(b) Reconstruction

17

Total Gastrectomy

(Roux–en–Y reconstruction)

Indications

Carcinoma of the stomach.

Operative details

The operation is performed through a thoracoabdominal incision by extending an upper abdominal incision through the line of the left eighth rib, giving access to the lower oesophagus. The whole stomach, together with the greater omentum and associated nodes, the spleen and sometimes the tail of the pancreas (*radical total gastrectomy*), are removed.

There are a number of options for restoring continuity. Shown here is a Roux–en–Y reconstruction in which the jejunum (b) is anastomosed to the lower oesophagus, while the fourth part of the duodenum (a) is anastomosed a further 50 cm downstream (c). (See Figure 6).

Notes

This method of reconstruction diverts bile and pancreatic secretions well down the jejunum, minimizing the risk of their reflux back up the oesophagus.

This Y – shaped reconstruction is often used in gastric surgery.

Roux was a Swiss surgeon.

Total Gastrectomy

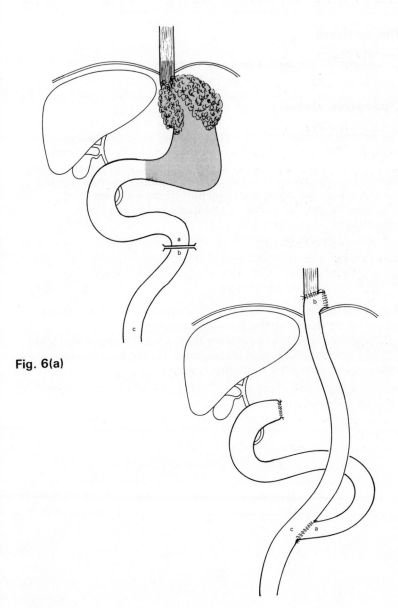

Fig. 6(a)

Fig. 6(b) Roux–en–Y reconstruction

Proximal Gastrectomy

Indications

Carcinoma of the cardia or body of stomach.

Operative details

The operation is performed through either an upper abdominal or a thoracoabdominal incision. The proximal stomach is removed with the tumour. The vagus nerves are taken with the specimen. The remaining stomach is formed into a tube by suturing along the line a-b-c. The most proximal part of the remnant (c-d), originally the greater curve, is anastomosed to the lower oesophagus. (See Figure 7).

A *pyloroplasty*, or *pyloromyotomy*, is performed.

Notes

A pyloroplasty is performed because cutting the vagus nerves results in paralysis of the pyloric sphincter.

This operation is less extensive than a total gastrectomy and so does not provide such a lasting cure. It may be preferred because the operative mortality is lower.

Proximal Gastrectomy

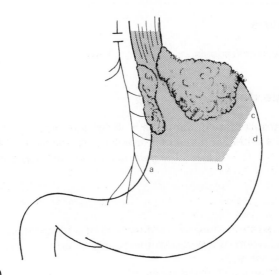

Fig. 7(a)

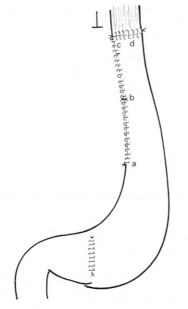

Fig. 7(b)   Reconstruction

Ramstedt's Pyloromyotomy

Indications

Infantile pyloric stenosis.

Operative details

The hypertrophied pyloric muscle is divided longitudinally, allowing the underlying mucosa to bulge into the split that has been created. This widens the pyloric canal. (See Figure 8).

Notes

A similar procedure may be used instead of a pyloroplasty following division of the vagi in the course of an *oesophagectomy*.
Ramstedt was a German surgeon.

Ramstedt's Pyloromyotomy

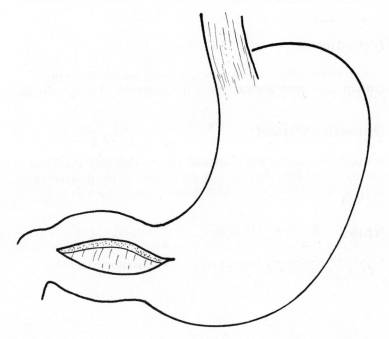

Fig. 8

Gastrojejunostomy

(Gastroenterostomy)

Indications

Pyloric obstruction, e.g. pyloric stenosis, carcinoma of the antrum. Duodenal obstruction, e.g. carcinoma of the pancreas.

Operative details

A loop of jejunum is anastomosed side-to-side onto the distal stomach. The loop may be brought up behind the transverse colon (retrocolic) or in front (antecolic). (See Figure 9).

Notes

A gastrojejunostomy forms part of the operation of a *Polya gastrectomy*.

24

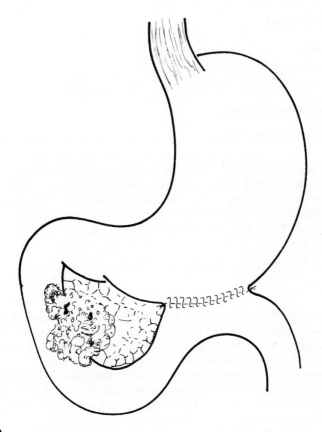

Fig. 9

BILIARY TRACT

Cholecystectomy

Indications

Gallstones.
Carcinoma of the gall bladder.

Operative details

The gall bladder and the stones it contains are removed. The cystic duct is ligated flush with the common bile duct.

During the procedure a cholangiogram is performed to determine whether any stones have escaped from the gall bladder and are lying within the common bile duct. Should this be the case, the common bile duct is opened and the stones extracted. The common bile duct is closed around a latex T-tube. (See Figure 10).

Notes

If stones within the common bile duct cannot be removed, then it may be necessary to extract them from below by means of a *transduodenal sphincteroplasty*. If this is too hazardous, then a *choledochoduodenostomy* is used to bypass them.

Following any surgery on the common bile duct, it is wise to leave a T-tube draining the duct to prevent any leakage of bile should the duct become obstructed by oedema and the pressure within it increase.

The T-tube is removed on the tenth postoperative day, provided that a further X-ray confirms that the common bile duct is clear of obstruction.

Cholecystectomy

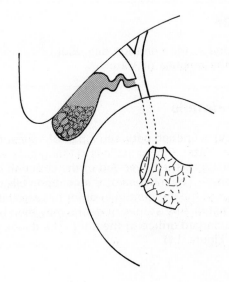

Fig. 10(a)

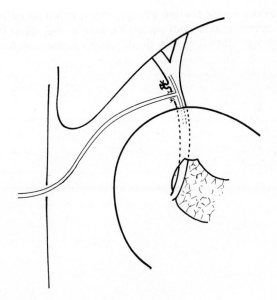

Fig. 10(b)   T-tube in common bile duct

Transduodenal Sphincteroplasty

Indications

Impacted stone in the common bile duct.
Stricture of the ampulla of Vater.

Operative details

The duodenum is opened between a pair of stay sutures opposite
the ampulla of Vater. The ampulla is slit longitudinally for
1–2 cm, opening up the lower end of the common bile duct
(sphincterotomy). The mucosa of the common bile duct is sewn
to the mucosa of the duodenum in order to keep the duct open
(sphincteroplasty). Any stones or debris may then be removed
through the enlarged orifice of the duct. The duodenum is then
closed. (See Figure 11).

Notes

The procedure is used when stones, etc. cannot be extracted
from the common bile duct via an incision in the upper duct
(exploration of common bile duct – see *cholecystectomy*).

Transduodenal Sphincteroplasty

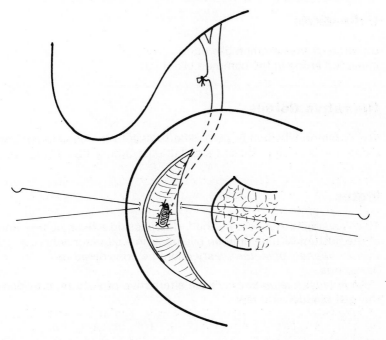

Fig. 11

29

Choledochoduodenostomy

Indications

Stricture of the common bile duct.
Impacted stone in the common bile duct.

Operative details

The common bile duct is sewn side-to-side to the duodenum. The stoma must be of sufficient size (at least 3 cm). (See Figure 12).

Notes

This is a simple and safe method of bypassing a fixed obstruction at the bottom of the common bile duct, in a situation where a *transduodenal sphincteroplasty* might be considered too hazardous.

A *cholecystojejunostomy* is an alternative procedure, provided the gall bladder is intact.

Choledochoduodenostomy

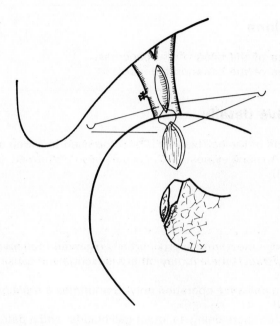

Fig. 12

Cholecystojejunostomy

Indications

Carcinoma of the head of the pancreas.
Carcinoma of the common bile duct.

Operative details

The fundus of the gall bladder is anastomosed to a loop of
jejunum. A jejunojejunostomy is usually also performed. (See
Figure 13).

Notes

The jejunojejunostomy diverts partially digested food away from
the biliary tract, where it may otherwise lodge and cause
infection.

This is a palliative operation only. Sometimes a *triple bypass* is
performed.

It relies on there being an intact gall bladder and a patent cystic
duct. *Choledochojejunostomy* is an alternative procedure in these
cases.

Cholecystojejunostomy

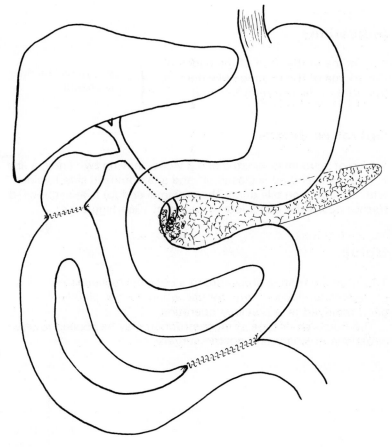

Fig. 13

Choledochojejunostomy

(Roux–en–Y reconstruction)

Indications

Carcinoma of the head of the pancreas
Carcinoma of the common bile duct
Stricture of the common bile duct
} – where gall bladder
is absent.

Operative details

A loop of jejunum is isolated and divided, leaving two ends, a and
b. The distal end (a) is closed off and anastomosed side-to-side
with the common bile duct. The proximal end (b) is anastomosed
further down the distal loop at point c. (See Figure 14).

Notes

This is an alternative procedure to a *cholecystojejunostomy* or a
choledochoduodenostomy, for use when the gall bladder has
been removed at a previous operation.

The Roux–en–Y type of reconstruction may be applied to other
situations in biliary and gastric surgery.

Choledochojejunostomy

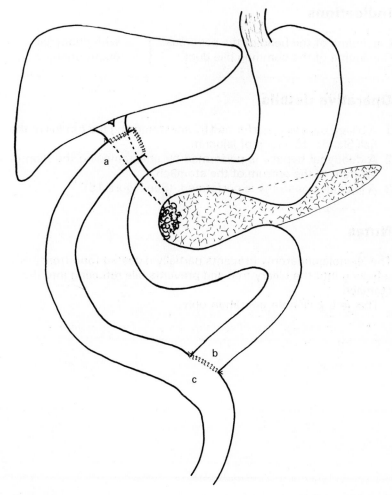

Fig. 14

Triple Bypass

Indications

Carcinoma of the head of the pancreas ⎫ – with duodenal
Carcinoma of the common bile duct ⎭   obstruction.

Operative details

1 A biliary bypass is performed by anastomosing the fundus of the
  gall bladder to a loop of jejunum.
2 A duodenal bypass is performed by anastomosing the loop of
  jejunum to the antrum of the stomach.
3 A jejunojejunostomy is performed. (See Figure 15).

Notes

The jejunojejunostomy prevents partially digested food from
refluxing into the biliary tree and prevents bile refluxing into the
stomach.
    This is a palliative operation only.

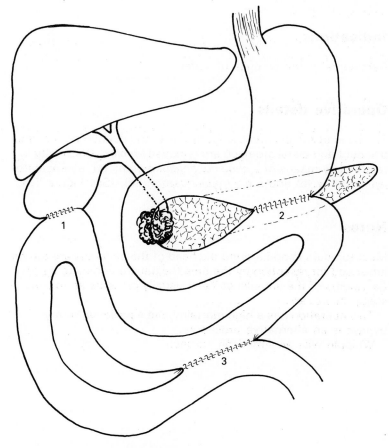

Fig. 15 1. Cholecystojejunostomy
2. Gastrojejunostomy
3. Jejunojejunostomy

Whipple's Operation
(Pancreatoduodenectomy)

Indications

Carcinoma of the ampulla of Vater.

Operative details

The head of the pancreas, together with the duodenum, common bile duct and distal stomach are removed *en bloc*. Continuity is restored by means of a *choledochojejunostomy* (a), a *pancreato-jejunostomy* (b) and a *gastrojejunostomy* (c). (See Figure 16).

Notes

Most tumours in and around the head of the pancreas are too far advanced for resection by the time the patient comes to surgery. Carcinoma of the ampulla of Vater usually presents at an early stage, however.

This operation has a high mortality and a palliative biliary bypass is an alternative procedure.

Whipple was an American surgeon.

Whipple's Operation

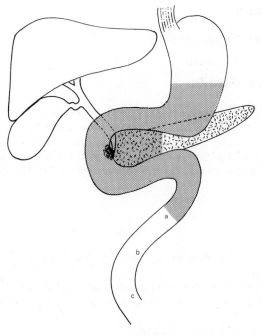

Fig. 16(a)   Pancreatoduodenectomy

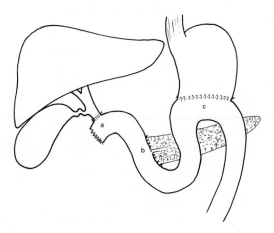

Fig. 16(b)   Reconstruction

OESOPHAGUS

Heller's Operation

Indications

Achalasia of the oesophagus.

Operative details

A longitudinal incision is made over the gastro-oesophageal junction, extending about 5 cm up the oesophagus and 5 cm onto the stomach. The incision divides the muscle coat, but not the underlying mucosa, which bulges into the slit. An anti-reflux procedure is sometimes performed, usually a *fundoplication*. (See Figure 17).

Notes

The operation is similar in technique to *Ramstedt's pyloromyotomy*.

Division of the muscle coat causes incompetence of the lower oesophageal sphincter mechanism, and may predispose to reflux of gastric acid.

Heller was a German surgeon.

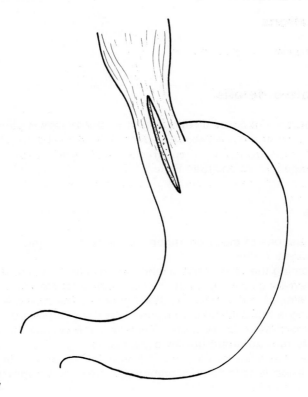

Fig. 17

Nissen Fundoplication

Indications

Hiatal hernia.

Operative details

The hiatus is tightened by approximating the stretched fibres of the left crus of the diaphragm around the lower oesophagus. The fundus of the stomach is then wrapped around the gastro-oesophageal junction. (See Figure 18).

Notes

This is just one of many operations for hiatal hernia and oesophageal reflux.

Tightening the crus of the diaphragm prevents the stomach from herniating into the chest – a condition predisposing to reflux. Wrapping the fundus of the stomach around the lower oesophagus (fundoplication) ensures that the oesophagus enters the stomach at an acute angle. This makes it less easy for gastric contents to regurgitate up the oesophagus.

Nissen was a Swiss surgeon. The repair of the diaphragm is not attributable to him and is common to most of the operations for hiatal hernia.

Nissen Fundoplication

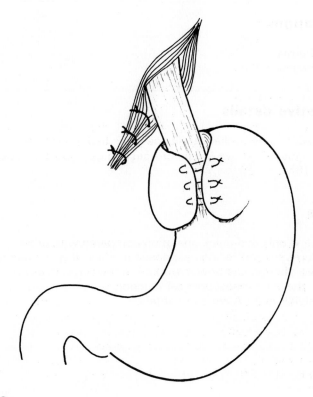

Fig. 18

Angelchik Prosthesis

Indications

Hiatal hernia.
Oesophageal reflux.

Operative details

A sausage-shaped collar of silicone gel is tied around the lower
oesophagus just above the gastro-oesophageal junction. (See
Figure 19).

Notes

This is a simple and quick operation compared with other
procedures for controlling oesophageal reflux. It is claimed to be
effective, though just how it works is not clear. It does *not*
narrow the gastro-oesophageal junction.
   Angelchik is an American surgeon.

44

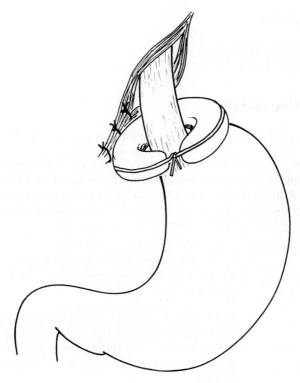

Fig. 19

Oesophagectomy

Indications

Carcinoma of the oesophagus.
Benign stricture of the oesophagus.

Operative details

The stomach is mobilized via an abdominal incision. A
pyloroplasty or a *pyloromyotomy* is performed (c).
　The abdomen is closed and a second incision made into the
right pleural cavity (right thoracotomy). The oesophagus is
mobilized and the stomach is drawn up into the pleural cavity.
The oesophagus is divided at the level of the gastro-oesophageal
junction, which is then closed with a suture (a).

Reconstruction:　*Ivor Lewis (2-stage procedure)*
　　　　　　　　The upper, intrathoracic oesophagus is
　　　　　　　　anastomosed to the highest part of the
　　　　　　　　stomach – the fundus (b).
　　　　　　　　McKeown (3-stage procedure)
　　　　　　　　The stomach is drawn through the pleural
　　　　　　　　cavity and on up into the neck where, through
　　　　　　　　a third incision, the fundus (b) is anastomosed
　　　　　　　　to the cervical oesophagus at the level of the
　　　　　　　　thyroid.

(See Figure 20).

Notes

After division of all but two of the arteries supplying it, the
stomach may be elongated so that it will reach up into the neck.
The vagus nerves are removed with the oesophagus, making a
pyloroplasty necessary to prevent gastric stasis (see *vagotomy
and pyloroplasty*).
　The 2-stage procedure is the shorter operation, but it is
technically more difficult to perform an anastomosis within the
pleural cavity. It is probably safer for the anastomosis to be in the
neck, in case it leaks.

Oesophagectomy

The second stage of the 3-stage procedure may be circumvented altogether in favourable circumstances, and the oesophageal resection performed by synchronous dissection through the abdominal and cervical incisions.

Lewis was a Welsh surgeon. McKeown is an English surgeon.

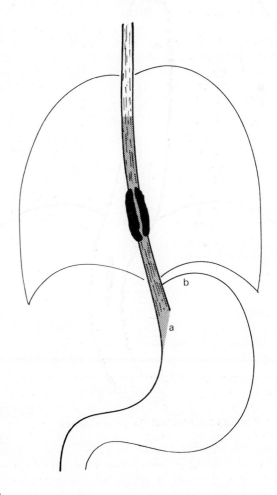

Fig. 20(a)

Oesophagectomy

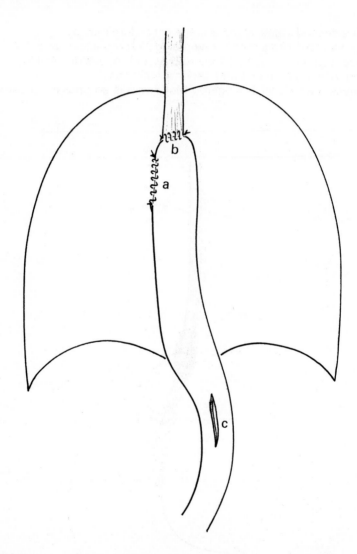

Fig. 20(b) 2-Stage reconstruction – Ivor Lewis

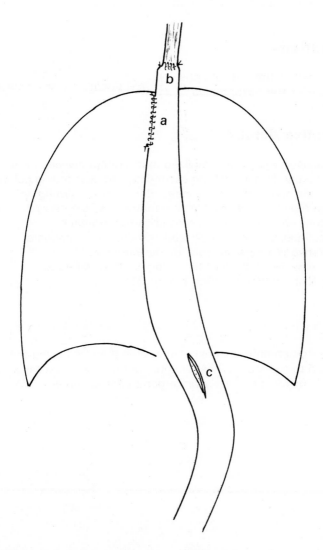

Fig. 20(c)   3-Stage reconstruction − McKeown

Oesophagectomy
(Colon interposition)

Indications

Carcinoma of the oesophagus
Stricture of the oesophagus } and previous gastric surgery.

Operative details

The transverse colon is mobilized, but without division of its blood supply. Division of the ascending and descending colon allows one end of the transverse colon (a) to be swung up through the chest where it is anastomosed to the oesophagus. The other end (b) is anastomosed to the stomach.

Sometimes the colon is passed into the neck through a subcutaneous tunnel in front of the sternum.

The remaining halves of the colon are then joined to re-establish continuity. (See Figure 21).

Notes

This is a much more extensive operation than that using the stomach to replace the oesophagus, but it may be necessary if the patient has previously undergone gastric surgery.

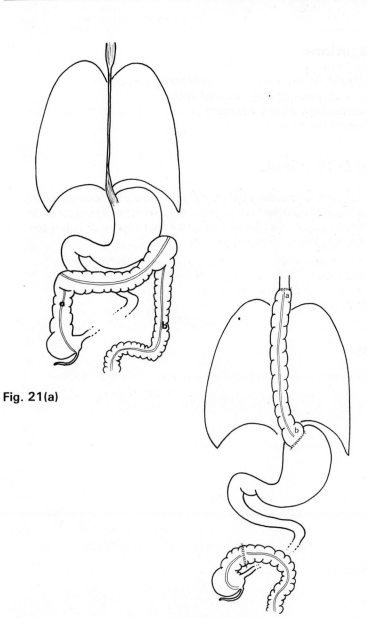

Fig. 21(a)

Fig. 21(b)   Reconstruction by colon interposition

COLORECTUM
Right Hemicolectomy

Indications

Carcinoma of the caecum or ascending colon.
Crohn's disease of the terminal ileum.
Angiodysplasia of the caecum.
Ileocaecal tuberculosis.

Operative details

The caecum, ascending colon and right side of transverse colon are removed together with a few centimetres of terminal ileum. Continuity is restored by end-to-end anastomosis of ileum to transverse colon. (See Figure 22).

Right Hemicolectomy

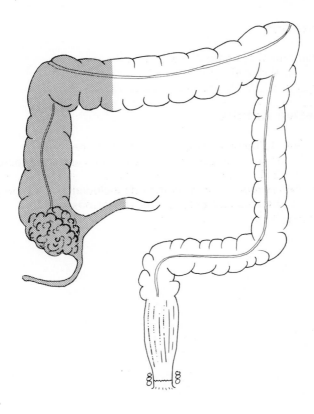

Fig. 22

Sigmoid Colectomy

Indications

Carcinoma of the sigmoid colon.
Diverticular disease.

Operative details

The sigmoid colon is removed and continuity restored by end-to-end anastomosis of the descending colon to the rectum. (See Figure 23).

A *transverse loop colostomy* may be included as a temporary measure to bypass and protect the anastomosis.

Sigmoid Colectomy

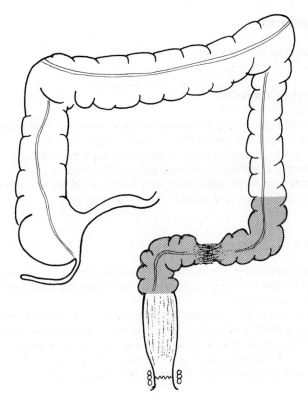

Fig. 23

Anterior Resection of the Rectum

Indications

Carcinoma of the rectum.

Operative details

The sigmoid colon and upper rectum are removed. Continuity is restored by anastomosing the descending colon to the remaining rectum. A staple gun is sometimes used to perform the anastomosis in difficult circumstances. (See Figure 24).

A *transverse loop-colostomy* may be included as a temporary measure to bypass and protect the anastomosis.

Notes

Anterior resection is performed through an abdominal incision, as opposed to the now outmoded approach from the sacral region (posterior resection).

Anterior resection may not be suitable for malignant tumours that arise within 5–6 cm of the anus, or those that involve the anal sphincters. In these circumstances the more radical procedure of *abdominoperineal resection*, in which the complete rectum and anal canal are removed, is to be preferred.

Anterior Resection of the Rectum

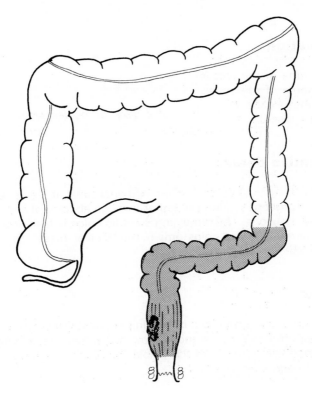

Fig. 24

Abdominoperineal Resection of the Rectum

Indications

Carcinoma of the rectum.
Carcinoma of the anus.
Ulcerative colitis ⎫
Crohn's disease   ⎬ – as part of a *panproctocolectomy*.

Operative details

The lower sigmoid colon, rectum and anal canal are removed by two surgeons working together through abdominal and perineal incisions. The remaining sigmoid colon is fashioned into a permanent end colostomy in the left iliac fossa. (See Figure 25).

Notes

Although an extensive and mutilating operation, it provides the best opportunity for clearance of low rectal tumours. When combined with removal of the whole colon, the procedure is termed *panproctocolectomy*.

Abdominoperineal Resection of the Rectum

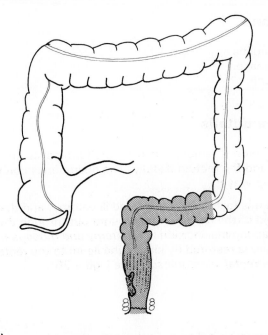

Fig. 25(a)

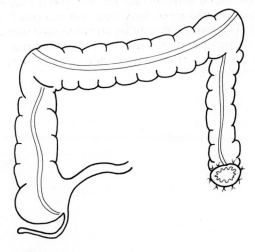

Fig. 25(b)   Completion

Total Colectomy

Indications

Ulcerative colitis.
Crohn's disease.
Polyposis coli.

Operative details

The whole colon is removed, leaving the terminal ileum proximally and the rectum distally. The operation is completed in either of two ways:

a) The ileum is fashioned into an end ileostomy, and the proximal end of the rectal stump brought out through the lower end of the abdominal incision – *ileostomy and mucous fistula*.
b) Continuity is restored by joining the ileum to the rectal stump – *ileorectal anastomosis*. (See Figure 26).

Notes

In severe ulcerative colitis or Crohn's disease, it is unwise to perform an ileorectal anastomosis for fear that it may not heal. The alternative procedure of *ileostomy and mucous fistula* is to be preferred. The two ends may be anastomosed and continuity restored at a later operation when the patient is fitter. If the condition of the rectal stump deteriorates, then it may have to be removed (*proctectomy*).

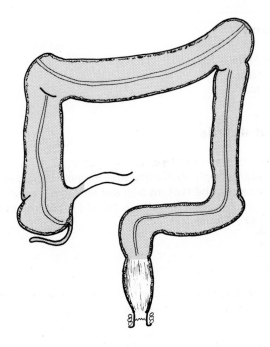

Fig. 26(a)

Fig. 26(b) Ileostomy and mucous fistula

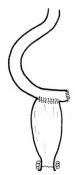

Fig. 26(c) Ileorectal anastomosis

Panproctocolectomy

Indications

Ulcerative colitis.
Crohn's disease.
Polyposis coli.

Operative details

The operation is performed by two surgeons working
synchronously through abdominal and perineal incisions. The
whole of the colon, the rectum and the anal canal are removed.
The terminal ileum is fashioned into an end ileostomy in the right
iliac fossa. (See Figure 27).

Notes

The procedure is similar to that of *abdominoperineal resection of
the rectum*, but is more extensive.

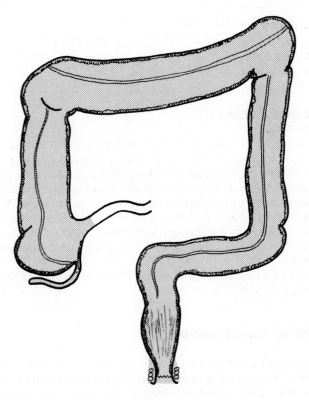

Fig. 27

Ileal Reservoir (Pouch)

Indications

Ulcerative colitis.
Polyposis coli.

Operative details

The diseased colon and the rectum, apart from a short rectal
stump, are removed, either at a previous operation or as a
prelude to forming the reservoir. Two, three or even four (as
shown here) loops of ileum are sutured together and the walls of
the loops opened out to form one big cavity. (See Figure 28). The
mucosa of the remaining rectum and anal canal is removed,
leaving a muscular tube through which the outlet of the reservoir
is drawn. The outlet is then sewn to the inside of the denuded
anal canal.

A temporary loop ileostomy is performed upstream of the
reservoir.

Details of construction

A reservoir formed from two loops of ileum is shown in Figure 29
for clarity. The loops are approximated by a continuous suture
and then the bowel is incised along its antimesenteric border (a).
This is shown in cross-section (b).

The cut edges of the bowel are sewn together so as to convert
the two adjacent loops into one big cavity (c).

Notes

This is a complex procedure and is used if the patient wishes
particularly to avoid a permanent ileostomy. It is not used in
Crohn's disease because of the possibility of recurrence of the
disease in the reservoir. The advantages over a straightforward
ileoanal anastomosis are that frequency of bowel actions is
reduced. Once the reservoir has healed, the loop ileostomy is
closed at a second operation.

Ileal Reservoir (Pouch)

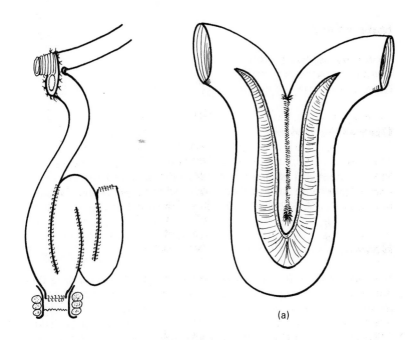

(a)

Fig. 28 Pouch and defunctioning loop ileostomy

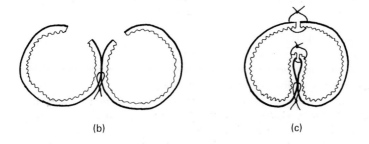

(b)   (c)

Fig. 29(a), (b), (c) Details of construction

Hartmann's Procedure

Indications

Perforated sigmoid colon.
Obstructed sigmoid colon.
Gangrenous sigmoid colon.

Operative details

The sigmoid colon is removed. Continuity is not restored initially.
The proximal end (descending colon) is fashioned into an
end colostomy in the left iliac fossa, and the distal end (rectum)
is oversewn. It is left *in situ*. (See Figure 30).

Notes

This operation is performed when it is necessary to remove the
colon, but too risky to perform an anastomosis because of the
presence of sepsis. Continuity may be restored at a later date
when the sepsis has been controlled and the patient is fitter.
  Sometimes the distal end is also fashioned into a stoma
(mucous fistula), which aids subsequent reconstruction.
  Hartmann was a French surgeon.

Hartmann's Procedure

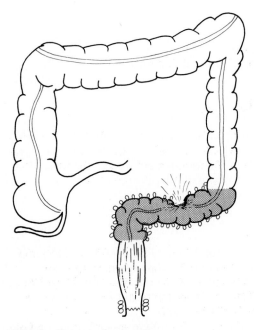

Fig. 30(a)   Extent of resection

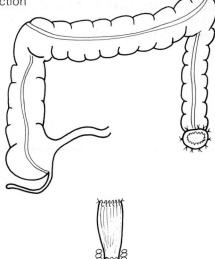

Fig. 30(b)   Completion

Transverse Loop Colostomy

Indications

Obstructed distal colon.
Protection of a distal colorectal anastomosis.

Operative details

The right side of the transverse colon is brought out through a
small incision and looped over a plastic or glass rod. The bowel is
opened at this point and the mucosa sutured to the skin. (See
Figure 31).

Notes

This quick and simple manœuvre may be used to deflate and
decompress an obstructed colon if the patient is too ill to
undergo any major resection of bowel. It may also be performed
as an adjunct to an *anterior resection* to act as a temporary
bypass while the anastomosis heals.

A loop colostomy may be performed at any point in the colon,
though the transverse colon is the most mobile.

This is usually a temporary procedure, and the colostomy is
closed at a later operation.

Transverse Loop Colostomy

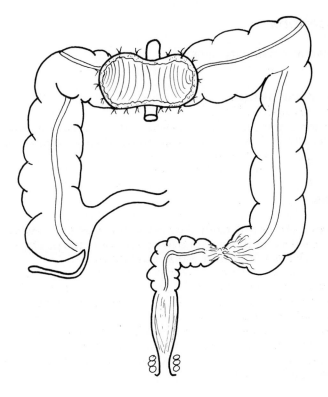

Fig. 31

Defunctioning End Colostomy

Indications

Unresectable pelvic malignancy.

Operative details

The colon is transected and, without resection, the proximal end is fashioned into a colostomy and the distal end oversewn. (See Figure 32).

Notes

This operation permanently diverts the faecal stream, making life more bearable for those with a fixed tumour in the pelvis, e.g. recurrent widespread rectal carcinoma.

Defunctioning End Colostomy

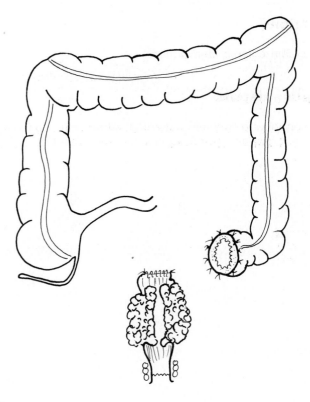

Fig. 32

Colocolostomy

Indications

Unresectable colonic obstruction.

Operative details

Two neighbouring segments of colon, either side of a fixed obstruction, are anastomosed side-to-side. (See Figure 33).

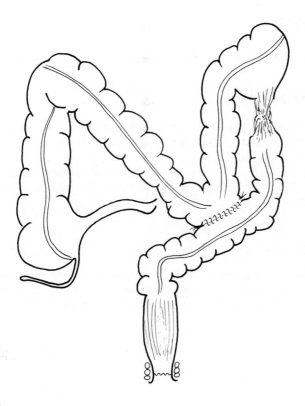

Fig. 33

Ivalon Sponge Rectopexy

Indications

Rectal prolapse.

Operative details

The rectum is mobilized from the pelvis and is enveloped in a sheet of polyvinyl alcohol sponge (Ivalon). The sponge is sewn to the muscle coat of the rectum, but it does not completely enclose the rectum for fear of causing obstruction. The sponge is then sewn to the sacrum, thus securing the rectum. (See Figure 34).

Notes

There are many operations for rectal prolapse. This is one of the more popular procedures and, although it is a major operation, the success rate is high compared with other methods.

Ivalon Sponge Rectopexy

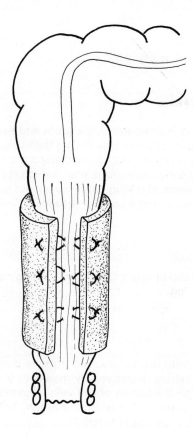

Fig. 34

BLOOD VESSELS
Femoropopliteal Bypass

Indications

Superficial femoral artery occlusion.

Operative details

The femoral artery is exposed in the groin and the popliteal artery exposed either just below or just above the knee, depending on the extent of the disease. The two incisions are then joined along the course of the long saphenous vein, which is removed. After clamping the arteries, the long saphenous vein is reversed and sewn to the femoral and popliteal arteries. (See Figure 35).

Notes

The vein is reversed in order that its valves may allow the flow of blood down the leg.

Variations

In-situ *vein*: The vein is not removed from its bed. Its branches are tied and the valves destroyed by means of a valve stripper passed up through the lumen of the vein. *Prosthetic graft:* If the vein is absent or too small, a graft of Dacron, Teflon or human umbilical vein may be substituted.

Femoropopliteal Bypass

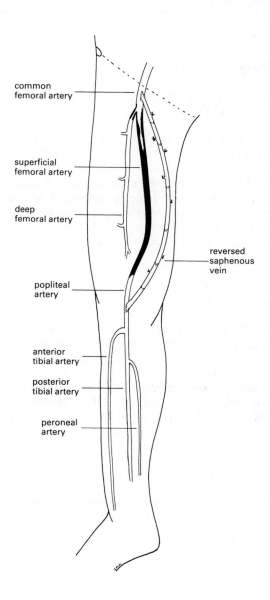

common
femoral artery

superficial
femoral artery

deep
femoral artery

reversed
saphenous
vein

popliteal
artery

anterior
tibial artery

posterior
tibial artery

peroneal
artery

Fig. 35

Profundaplasty

(Endarterectomy)

Indications

Stenosis of the origin of the profunda femoris (deep femoral) artery.

Operative details

The common femoral artery is exposed at its bifurcation into the superficial and the profunda femoris arteries. After clamping the arteries, an incision is made into the profunda femoris. Atheroma from within the artery is removed. The incision is closed by inlaying a patch of saphenous vein or Dacron. (See Figure 36).

Notes

This procedure is performed when the profunda femoris is the only patent vessel supplying the leg. It is often combined with a more proximal procedure such as an *aortobifemoral graft*. Using a patch to close the incision acts as a gusset, enlarging the lumen of the artery.

Profundaplasty is an example of the procedure of end-arterectomy which may be applied to short stenoses in other arteries, e.g. internal carotid, aorta, iliac.

Profundaplasty

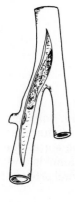

1. Incision into artery

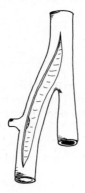

2. Removal of atheroma

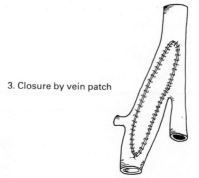

3. Closure by vein patch

Fig. 36　1.　Incision into artery
　　　　　　2.　Removal of atheroma
　　　　　　3.　Closure by vein patch

Aortobifemoral Graft

Indications

Stenosis or occlusion of the iliac arteries.

Operative details

A laparotomy is performed and the aorta clamped. Both femoral arteries in the groins are exposed and clamped. A bifurcated Dacron graft is sewn onto the anterior wall of the aorta. The limbs of the graft are passed into the groins via tunnels under the inguinal ligament. Each limb is sewn onto a femoral artery. (See Figure 37).

Notes

If the disease does not affect the external iliac arteries, an aortoiliac graft may be performed. This is performed entirely within the abdomen, obviating the need for separate groin incisions.

Aortobifemoral Graft

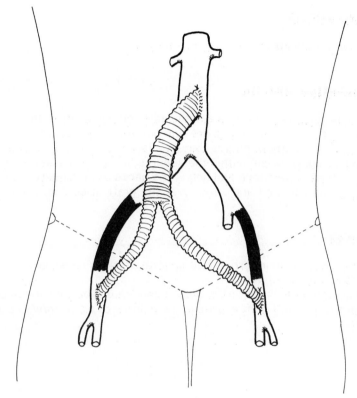

Fig. 37

81

Aortic Aneurysm Repair

Indications

Aortic aneurysm.

Operative details

A laparotomy is performed and the aorta clamped above the aneurysm. The iliac arteries are clamped below it. The aneurysm is opened and the thrombus that it usually contains is removed. A Dacron graft is laid within the aneurysmal sac and is sewn to the normal aorta above and below the necks of the aneurysm. The sac is trimmed and sewn over the graft. (See Figure 38).

Notes

The graft is inlaid into the existing aorta. It is not necessary to remove the aneurysm.

The common iliac arteries may be aneurysmal as well, in which case a bifurcated graft is used in the manner of an *aortobifemoral graft*.

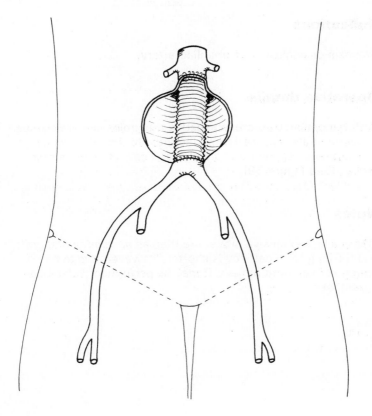

Fig. 38

Femorofemoral Cross-Over Graft

Indications

Stenosis or occlusion of one iliac artery.

Operative details

Both femoral arteries are exposed in the groins and are clamped. A Dacron graft is passed from one groin to the other via a subcutaneous suprapubic tunnel and is sewn to each femoral artery. (See Figure 39).

Notes

This is a less extensive procedure than an *aortobifemoral graft* and the long-term patency is shorter. However, it is to be preferred in an unfit patient. It may be performed under local anaesthetic.

Femorofemoral Cross-Over Graft

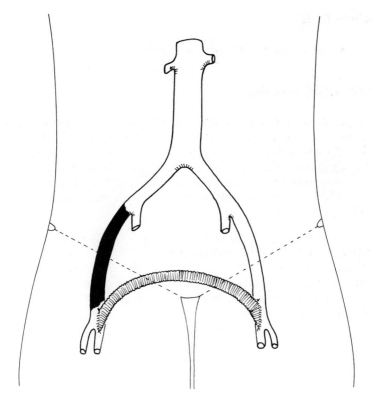

Fig. 39

Axillobifemoral Graft

Indications

Stenosis or occlusion of both iliac arteries.

Operative details

The axillary artery is exposed just below the middle of the clavicle, and the femoral arteries exposed in each groin. After clamping the arteries, a bifurcated Dacron graft is tunnelled subcutaneously from each incision. A further incision in the flank is made to assist the creation of the long tunnel from axilla to groin. The limbs of the graft are sewn to their respective arteries. (See Figure 40).

Notes

This is a less extensive procedure than an *aortobifemoral graft* and the long-term patency is shorter. However, it is to be preferred in an unfit patient.

Axillobifemoral Graft

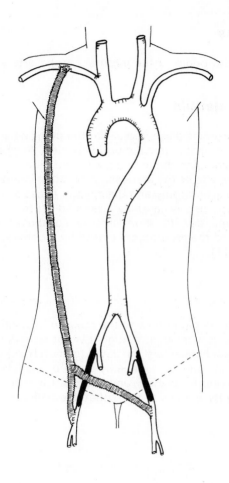

Fig. 40

Carotid Endarterectomy

Indications

Stenosis of the origin of the internal carotid artery.

Operative details

The carotid artery is dissected out at the point where it divides into the internal and external carotid arteries. After administering heparin and clamping the arteries, a longitudinal arteriotomy is made over the site of the stenosis. A shunt is inserted into the artery via the arteriotomy and the clamps released. Atheroma causing the stenosis is carefully dissected off the inside of the artery and removed. The shunt is removed, the arteries briefly re-clamped and the arteriotomy closed by a continuous suture. (See Figure 41).

Notes

The shunt allows blood flow to the brain to be maintained during the time the artery is open, though it is not always used. The two shunts commonly used are the Javid (shown here) which is a simple tube held snugly in place by a pair of ring clamps (omitted from the drawing for clarity), and the Pruitt-Inahara which is self-retaining by means of two inflatable balloons.

Carotid Endarterectomy

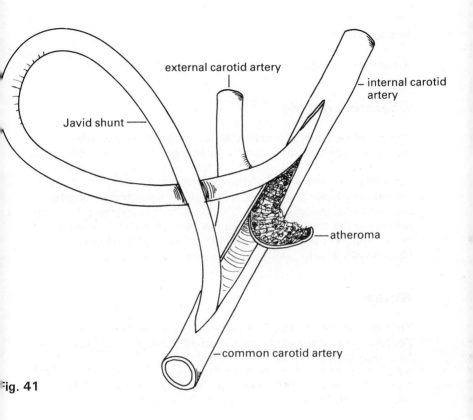

external carotid artery

internal carotid artery

Javid shunt

atheroma

common carotid artery

Fig. 41

89

Embolectomy

Indications

Arterial embolism.

Operative details

The affected artery is exposed at a convenient site above or below the point of occlusion. Common sites include the femoral artery in the groin, the popliteal artery behind the knee and the brachial artery in the arm. After clamping the artery, an arteriotomy is performed and a Fogarty embolectomy catheter passed down the artery through the soft occluding embolus. The balloon at the end of the catheter is inflated and the catheter withdrawn, extracting the embolus with it. The arteriotomy is closed with a continuous suture. (See Figure 42).

Notes

This operation is often performed under local anaesthetic. Fogarty is an American surgeon and designed the catheter while he was a student.

Embolectomy

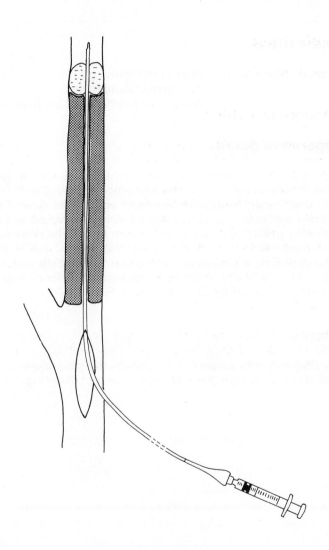

Fig. 42

URINARY TRACT
Ileal Conduit

Indications

Urinary diversion, e.g. after cystectomy.
                    neurogenic bladder.
                    congenital anomalies of bladder.

Operative details

About 20 cm of ileum is disconnected from the rest of the small
bowel, retaining its mesentery and blood supply. Continuity of
the small bowel is restored by end-to-end anastomosis. The two
ureters are mobilized, disconnected from the bladder and sewn
together to form one opening. The junction of the ureters is then
anastomosed to the proximal end of the isolated ileal segment. A
fine-bore tube is passed up each ureter to splint the anastom-
oses. The distal end of the ileal segment is fashioned into an end
ileostomy in the right iliac fossa. (See Figure 43).

Notes

Cystectomy may be performed prior to this procedure, if
indicated. There are many other methods of diverting the urine.

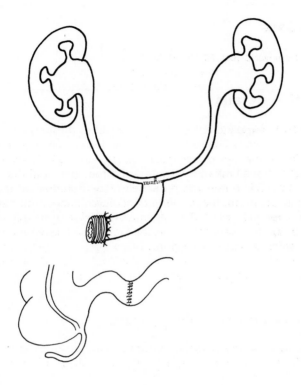

Fig. 43

Anderson–Hynes Pyeloplasty

Indications

Pelviureteric junction obstruction.

Operative details

The kidney is exposed either through a loin or through an abdominal incision. The redundant renal pelvis is excised (a-b-c) together with the obstructed pelviureteric junction. Aberrant vessels may have kinked the ureter, and they need careful preservation. The remaining renal pelvis is sutured along the line a-b. The upper ureter is *spatulated* and sewn back on to the opening in the pelvis b-c. This anastomosis is usually splinted by passing a fine-bore tube through the kidney and down the ureter (nephrostomy tube). (See Figure 44).

Notes

Anderson and Hynes are British surgeons.

Anderson–Hynes Pyeloplasty

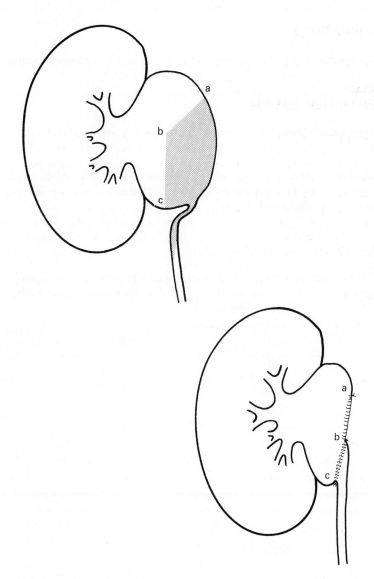

Fig. 44

Caecocystoplasty

Indications

Contracted bladder, e.g. tuberculosis, bilharzia, radiation cystitis.

Operative details

The caecum is isolated with its blood supply intact and disconnected from the terminal ileum and ascending colon. The appendix is removed. The caecum is turned upside down and anastomosed to the opened-out bladder. Continuity of the bowel is restored by end-to-end anastomosis of the ileum to ascending colon. (See Figure 45).

Notes

This procedure enlarges the capacity of a bladder that has been shrunk by disease. An isolated loop of ileum may be used in the same way – ileocystoplasty.

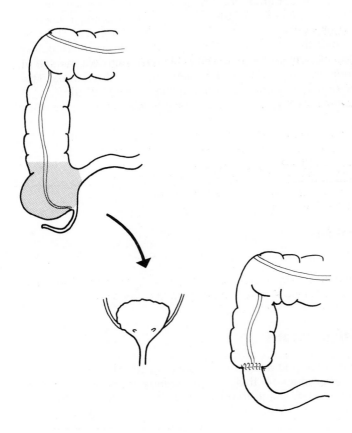

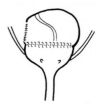

Fig. 45 Reconstruction

GENERAL

Anatomy of a Hernia

The sites of the common abdominal wall hernias are shown opposite. The principles of the anatomy are the same in each case though obviously there are individual differences. There is a protrusion of the peritoneum through a natural gap or weakness in the muscle wall of the abdomen. This gap narrows the *sac* of peritoneum into a *neck* before it opens out into the *fundus*. The sac may or may not contain some of the contents of the peritoneal cavity, e.g. omentum, small bowel. (See Figure 46(a)).

Repair of a Hernia

Indications

Pain.
Strangulation.
Obstruction.

Operative details

The sac is dissected out from surrounding structures. The contents are reduced if this has not already occurred. The sac is usually opened to check that the contents have been reduced and then it is transfixed, ligated and removed (herniotomy). The defect in the abdominal wall is repaired by approximating its edges, darning it or patching it using unabsorbable materials (herniorrhaphy).

Repair of a Hernia

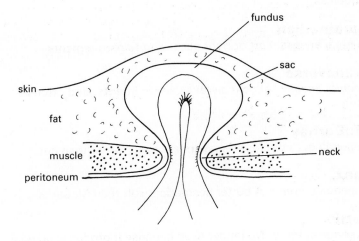

Fig. 46(a)

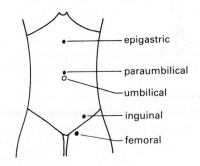

Fig. 46(b)   Common hernia sites

Incisions

(See Figure 47).

Midline
General access. Usually skirts the umbilicus. Quick and bloodless.

Paramedian
General access. Left or right according to requirements.

Transverse
General access. Almost always used in infants, and often in adults.

McBurney
Appendicectomy. Muscle layers are split, rather than cut.

Lanz
Appendicectomy. A better cosmetic result than McBurney.

Battle
Appendicectomy. No longer used because it produces an ugly scar and sometimes incisional hernia. Often seen in older patients therefore.

Kocher
Biliary or hepatic procedures. May be extended across to a left subcostal incision to give useful access to the stomach and pancreas.

Pfannenstiel
Access to bladder, uterus, Fallopian tubes and ovaries. Good cosmetic result but gives no access outside the pelvis.

Rutherford Morison
Access to sigmoid colon and pelvis, particularly if the midline is very scarred from previous surgery.

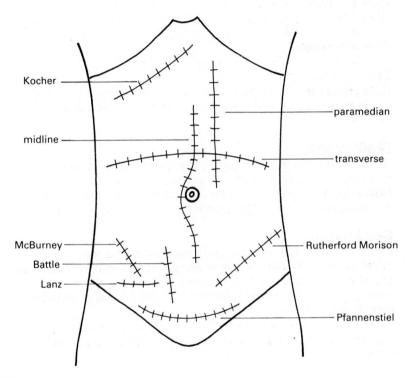

Fig. 47

Anastomoses

(See Figure 48).

End-to-end
Used when the two ends of bowel are of approximately the same diameter and there is no danger of stricture or of making the stoma too small.

End-to-side
Used when there is a discrepancy between the diameters of the two ends of bowel. An alternative is to use a *side-to-side* anastomosis.

Side-to-side
Used when there is a discrepancy between the diameters of the two ends of bowel. A stoma of any size may be constructed by this method. Often used to join two segments of bowel without resecting them, e.g. in obstruction.

Spatulated
Used for ureter and small blood vessels when it is important to avoid narrowing of the stoma in an end-to-end anastomosis. The free ends of each vessel are slit longitudinally for a few millimetres in order to open them out. They are then sutured to each other forming an oblique stoma.

Anastomoses

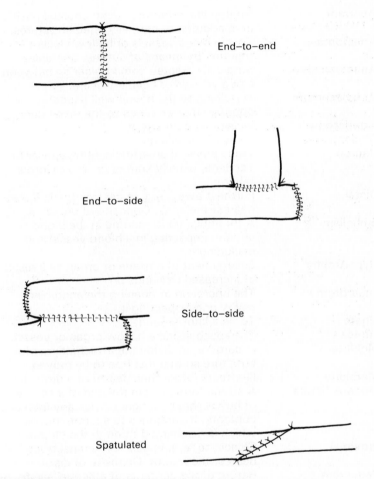

End–to–end

End–to–side

Side–to–side

Spatulated

Fig. 48

Glossary

Aberrant   Anatomical structures in an unusual position or in addition to normally-sited structures.

Anastomose   To join blood vessels or hollow viscera together by means of sutures or staples.

Anastomosis   Surgically created communication between blood vessels or hollow viscera.

Antimesenteric   Pertaining to the bowel wall diametrically opposite that attached to the mesentery.

Arteriotomy   Incision into an artery.

Cholangiogram   X-ray of the bile duct.

Dacron   Trade name of an artificial fibre, similar to Terylene, usually knitted or woven into a fabric.

Distal   Furthest away, e.g. in gastrointestinal tract, nearest the anus. Opposite of proximal.

Embolism   A thrombus (clot), carried in the blood stream, impacting in a blood vessel and occluding it.

Hypertrophy   Enlargement of a tissue or organ as a result of increased demands on it.

Laparotomy   The operation of opening the abdominal cavity and inspecting it.

Ligate   To tie a knot around.

Lumen   The space inside a hollow organ or vessel.

Mobilize   In surgery, to divide the attachments of a structure so that it is free to be moved.

Morbidity   Ill-effects (other than death) of a procedure.

Mucous fistula   A stoma formed from the end of a segment of bowel that no longer carries any intestinal contents. It continues to secrete mucus which is discharged through the stoma.

Proximal   Closest to, e.g. in gastrointestinal tract, nearest the mouth. Opposite of distal.

Reduction (of a hernia)   Return of the contents of a hernial sac to the peritoneal cavity.

Reflux   Backward flow.

Resection   Surgical removal.

Stenosis   Narrowing, but not complete occlusion.

Stoma   1. The orifice of an anastomosis.
2. Surgically created opening between the bowel and the skin of the abdomen.

Suture   Stitch.

Teflon   Trade name for tetrafluoroethylene.